Nought to — becoming me

A guide for parents (and those who support them)

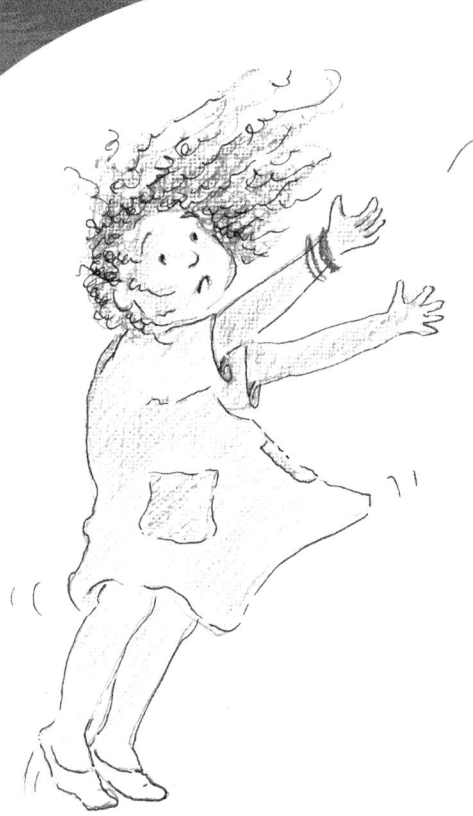

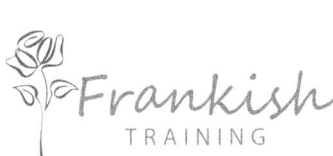

by Dr Pat Frankish

Nought to Three – Becoming Me

A guide for parents (and those who support them)

© Pavilion Publishing and Media Ltd

The author has asserted her rights in accordance with the Copyright, Designs and Patents Act (1988) to be identified as the author of this work.

Published by:
Pavilion Publishing and Media Ltd
Blue Sky Offices Shoreham
25 Cecil Pashley Way
Shoreham-by-Sea
West Sussex
BN43 5FF
Tel: 01273 434 943
Fax: 01273 227 308
Email: info@pavpub.com

Published 2019

All rights reserved. No part of this publication may be reproduced, stored in a retrieval system, or transmitted in any form or by any means, electronic, mechanical, photocopying, recording or otherwise, without prior permission in writing of the publisher and the copyright owners.

A catalogue record for this book is available from the British Library.

ISBN: 978-1-912755-80-6

Pavilion Publishing and Media is a leading publisher of books, training materials and digital content in mental health, social care and allied fields. Pavilion and its imprints offer must-have knowledge and innovative learning solutions underpinned by sound research and professional values.

Editor: Mike Benge, Pavilion Publishing and Media Ltd.
Cover design: Emma Dawe, Pavilion Publishing and Media Ltd.
Page layout and typesetting: Emma Dawe, Pavilion Publishing and Media Ltd.
Illustrations: Jo Hathaway
Printing: Severn Print

Contents

Acknowledgements v
Foreword vii

Chapter 1:
The Emotional Journey 1

Chapter 2:
Arriving in the World – Establishing the Symbiotic Relationship 7

Chapter 3:
Feeling Their Way – Differentiation 15

Chapter 4:
Learning Fast – Practising 19

Chapter 5:
Give and Take – Early Rapprochement 23

Chapter 6:
Moving Away – Late Rapprochement 27

Chapter 7:
Knowing Me, Knowing You – Making it to Individuation 31

Chapter 8:
Finding Support – What Happens When Things Go Wrong? 33

Epilogue:
Some Words of Reassurance 37

References 39

The publication you are reading is one of a series of titles created by Dr Pat Frankish for those supporting children and adults who have experienced trauma, particularly those with intellectual disabilities (learning disabilities).

Currently, the series includes:

Trauma-informed Care in Intellectual Disability: A self-study guide for health and social care support staff

Frankish Assessment of the Impact of Trauma in Intellectual Disability (FAIT)

Nought to Three – Becoming Me: A guide for parents (and those who support them)

For full information go to www.pavpub.com/nought-to-three-becoming-me

For Pat Frankish Training go to www.frankishtraining.co.uk

Acknowledgements

I have learned so much from the people I have worked with and known for the whole of my life, and particularly since I became a psychologist in 1985. It has been a joy to help people who seemed beyond help. It is a joy to see someone who is very withdrawn take an interest in another person. It has become so clear that trauma before age 3 or 4 is life changing and it will be good to see if we can make a difference.

Foreword

'It is easier to build strong children than to repair broken adults.'
F. Douglas

This book is about laying the foundations for your child to develop a core self that will take them through the rest of their lives. The ideas come from many years of working with people for whom this has not happened. If there is a way to enable small children to have better foundations to their personality it seems right to try. There is no hard research to back this up as it is not possible, or ethical, to deny one group of children in order to make a comparison. We will always have to use data from those for whom things have gone wrong.

Over my long career I have found many distressed people who have, ostensibly, had a good supportive family and yet have become mentally unwell or criminal and there is, inevitably, puzzlement about how this could have happened. I have also encountered many who have had a less than perfect start, some of whom have done well, and others who haven't. We know from research that children who have obvious traumatic life events have poorer outcomes. There is a question for me about the factors that lead to resilience and those that lead to distress. Another question is about the manifestation of that distress – is it serious mental health decline into psychosis, or depression, addiction, personality disorder, criminality, serious self-harm, autism, or a general feeling of malaise, of not being who you thought you were?

My own experience tells me that the people I meet clinically, including a wide range of people with disabilities and other psychological issues, can trace their distress back to early childhood. Perhaps the most poignant factor is that what they found traumatic was idiosyncratic, not necessarily something that others would recognise as traumatic, so the impact can be missed. Children are not born as a blank sheet; their interaction with the world is what matters, and no two are the same. This uniqueness is both a gift in that it leads to huge diversity, but can also make it very hard work to prescribe a way of raising children that will work for all.

An attempt is going to be made in this book to provide some ideas of how to help your child develop a secure sense of self, as well as how to recognise when there might be a hiccup and what to do to rectify the effect. I do know from therapeutic work that there can be recovery once the issues are identified, and that there can't be if they are not.

My aim is to be positive and helpful. Many parents blame themselves when things go wrong. Many children blame their parents. It is an interaction with multiple factors. Sometimes I think it is a miracle that any of us grows up sane and resilient. But clearly we do, so some things work out fine; the complexity of the process makes sure that we are all different, all unique, including identical twins, and that makes for the richness of human life.

This work is underpinned by that of Margaret Mahler and her colleagues. The findings explained in their book, *The Psychological Birth of the Human Infant* (1975), have influenced my own studies. They describe observable stages of emotional development from biological birth to the point of having a separate identity which she calls 'psychological birth'. I noticed the behaviours she described in children, also observable in adults with learning disabilities, and raised the question as to whether their distressed behaviour could be as a result of their emotional issues rather than their mental impairment. This has been shown to be the case. Since discovering this I have applied the theory to a wider range of people and found it to be the case that most distressed people can identify trauma in that period from biological to psychological birth. Their presentation is different from those who have experienced trauma in later life, after initially establishing a secure sense of self. Mahler refers to it as 'individuation', that state of being able to be separate from the primary caregiver with manageable anxiety. People who have trauma before individuation and then more trauma after that period will be the most distressed that we see.

The core issue is always about the availability of a safe and trusted significant other throughout this formative time. This does not have to be the same person 24 hours a day and seven days a week, but anyone 'caretaking' must be trusted, and seen to be trusted, by the significant other, and returning to the key person must be within the timeframe that the individual child can tolerate. If there are events that prevent this, the trajectory of development will be changed. Often this is not permanently harmful but it may lead to permanent changes that can be predicted to some extent, and can be recovered from if identified.

Chapter 1: The Emotional Journey

Mahler's stages of development

In 1975, Margaret Mahler and her colleagues wrote up the findings from their studies of the different stages of emotional development that they had observed in young children. In their book *The Psychological Birth of the Human Infant* they describe these stages, from biological birth to the point of the child having a separate identity, which Mahler described as 'psychological birth'.

The five stages they identified were:

- Symbiosis
- Differentiation
- Practising
- Rapprochement – early rapprochement and late rapprochement
- Individuation

Let's look at those in more detail – you may well recognise your own child, or children you know, in the behaviour described.

The road to individuation

Symbiotic
- age: newborn, first few weeks of life
- as if the mother and child still connected
- mother and child in very close enmeshed symbiotic relationship
- child is entirely dependent on the mother to have all its needs met

Differentiating
- age: a few weeks to about nine months
- baby develops an awareness of itself and the parts of its body
- baby looks at and plays with hands, feet and sometimes genitals
- become aware of their immediate surroundings, such as cot or pram, toys
- baby is only aware of a very small space around it
- 'self-referenced behaviours'
- baby only aware of other people being around, in terms of getting its own needs met

Practising
- age: approx 9–15 months
- baby becomes able to do new things on a very regular basis and starts to 'practise' new skills eg throwing rattle from pram, rolling over etc
- baby practises new skill again and again until it can do it well then moves on to another
- very important in the practising stage that someone is around watching and paying attention to the child – if baby is not watched/engaged they practise less, and learning slows

Rapprochement
- age: approx. 15 months to 3.5 years
- 'give and take' stage – child develops ability to have two-way, reciprocal, relationship with primary carers.

Early rapprochement
- age: approx. 15 months to 2 years
- child begins to learn to give and take
- child begins to say 'no', or walks away, showing start of two-way negotiation
- can be challenging for the parents – sometimes called the 'terrible twos'
- play is 'peek-a-boo' or 'round and round the garden' games about two-way communication

Late rapprochement
- age: approx. 2 years to 3.5 years
- negotiating and demanding to have needs met
- child gradually begins to increase the distance it can be away from the primary carers/parents
- manageable anxiety about separation – step by step
- 'emotional refuelling' is important in this stage to help the child feel confident
- growing confidence to move away from the carer to explore

Individuation
- the point where the child can be separate from the primary carer with manageable (not no) anxiety
- some children reach the individuation stage through a 'rapprochement crisis'
- the point of 'psychological birth' – child has reached sense of own identity, separate from parents, psychologically able to grow further into an independent human being

Symbiotic stage
The symbiotic stage is the newborn phase in the first few weeks of life. At this stage it is as if the mother and baby are still connected, still very close, and are in what Mahler described as an 'enmeshed' relationship, still feeling like 'one' body, as they were before birth. This relationship is called the symbiotic relationship. In the symbiotic stage the child is entirely dependent on its mother to have all his/her needs met.

Differentiation stage
The differentiation stage is when the baby develops an awareness of itself and the parts of its body. This stage starts at a few weeks and goes to about nine months. At this stage babies will look at and play with their hands, feet and sometimes their genitals. They also become aware of their immediate surroundings, such as the cot or pram that they are in, and the toys that are around them. At this stage the baby is only aware of a very small space around it and is beginning to notice that it exists within this small space.

The behaviours seen in the differentiation stage are called 'self-referenced behaviours'. This means that everything the baby does is about, or in reference to, itself. It doesn't do anything to influence anybody else. Although if the baby screams or cries this will influence others, the reason the baby does it is because it wants something for itself, that is, it is hungry or cold. The baby therefore is only aware of other people being around in terms of getting its own needs met.

Practising stage
Brain development in babies happens very quickly. Through this rapid brain development the baby becomes able to do new things on a very regular basis. Mahler and her colleagues found that a baby will start to 'practise' a new skill as it becomes available. The baby will practise the new skill again and again until it can do it well. So there is a developmental reason your baby throws the rattle out of the pram again and again – it isn't just to make you bend down and pick it up! Other behaviours would be learning to roll over, crawling and standing up.

> "...the baby will start to 'practise' a new skill as it becomes available. The baby will practise the new skill again and again until it can do it well. So there is a developmental reason your baby throws the rattle out of the pram again and again – it isn't just to make you bend down and pick it up!

This stage begins at around nine months and continues to around 15 months. The baby may practise behaviours at other times but this is the main practising stage. When the child can do a particular behaviour well, another becomes available due to the brain's rapid development. The child then begins practising this new behaviour.

It is very important in the practising stage that someone is around watching and paying attention to the child. Mahler found that if the child knew it was being watched, then the practising behaviour continued. If the child thought that nobody was paying attention they practised much less. This made learning a new behaviour much slower.

Rapprochement stage

The word rapprochement means 'give and take'. Give and take is one of the most important skills needed in relationships. In this stage the child is beginning to have a two-way, or reciprocal, relationship with its primary carers. This stage is divided into two sub-stages – early rapprochement, and late rapprochement. It goes from about 15 months to about three and a half years.

Early rapprochement

The early rapprochement stage is the start of the child beginning to learn to give and take. This begins around 15 months and goes on until about two years. The first sign that a child has moved into the early rapprochement stage is when the child begins to say 'no', or walks away. This shows the start of two-way negotiation. The child moving into this stage can be challenging for the parents. It is sometimes called the 'terrible twos'.

In this stage the child will become interested in 'peek-a-boo' or 'round and round the garden' games. These games are about two-way communication and give and take between two people.

Late rapprochement

The late rapprochement stage is the beginning of the child moving towards independence. This stage can be more challenging as the child is negotiating and can be demanding in getting its needs met. This happens from two to three years.

In this stage the child also gradually begins to increase the distance it can be away from the primary carers or parents. It can do this with its levels of anxiety being manageable. This is similar to the ideas of Winnicott (1964) and Bowlby (1988), who talked about the child gradually having the confidence to move away from the mother or 'safe base' and explore the world.

It is really important that the child's anxiety is manageable so they are not overwhelmed. Independence grows in small steps that the child can cope with. For example, at play group the child may start off being sat by its mother's feet. When it is a few months older the child will move away to play with the other children in the middle of the floor. It can do this by being able to keep an eye on mum and where she is. As the child moves into late rapprochement, it will be able to go a bit further away from mum. It can do this without being anxious about where she is.

> **'Emotional refuelling' is important in this stage to help the child feel confident. This is where the child will look round for the parent and make eye contact. This eye contact will 'emotionally refuel' the child and help them feel confident. They can then happily carry on playing at a distance from the carer.**

'Emotional refuelling' is important in this stage to help the child feel confident. This is where the child will look round for the parent and make eye contact. This eye contact will 'emotionally refuel' the child and help them feel confident. They can then happily carry on playing at a distance from the carer.

By having the confidence to move away from the carer, the child can begin to explore. Through this the child is learning about the world around it. The child is also beginning to understand its own place in the world.

Individuation stage

Once the child has moved fairly smoothly through the stages above it reaches the individuation stage. This is the point where the child can be separate from the primary carer with manageable anxiety. Note: this is not a state of having no anxiety. It is normal and indeed sometimes helpful to have some manageable anxiety. It is a state of not being overwhelmed by anxiety when separated from the parent or primary carer.

Some children reach the individuation stage through a 'rapprochement crisis'. This is when they realise the primary carer is not there, they become anxious, distressed and may have a tantrum. They then realise that they can cope with the situation. Individuation is the point of the child knowing that they are separate from the carer but that they can manage the anxiety of this.

Reaching the individuation stage is the 'psychological birth' of the child. It is the point that they have reached their own identity, as being separate from their parents. At this point the child is psychologically able to grow further into an independent human being, who can stand on their own two feet.

Chapter 1: The Emotional Journey

Margaret Mahler helps us to understand the stages that a child goes through to reach individuation. She helps us to know what behaviours can be seen at each stage. It is therefore possible, by observing the behaviour of a child, to work out what stage of emotional development they are at.

STOP AND THINK

about a child you know and relate the information you have just read to them. Think about how their behaviours changed as they went through the stages.

Chapter 2: Arriving in the World – Establishing the Symbiotic Relationship

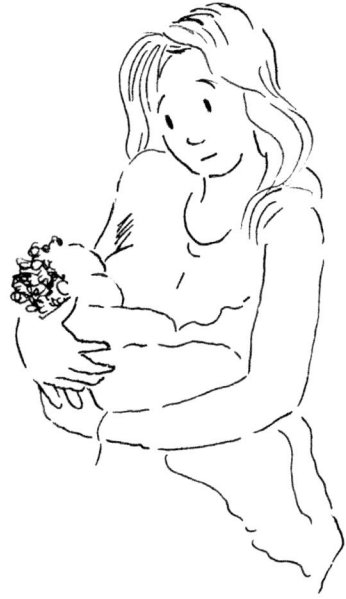

'The most important period of life is not the age of university studies, but the first one, the period from birth to the age of six.'
Maria Montessori

Biological birth – how your baby arrives in the world

Being born is a natural biological process, but it can have its hazards. It's not an easy thing to contemplate, especially if you are reading this just before it is due to happen. Many people aim to have a 'natural birth' and current antenatal practice encourages mothers to make positive choices about the way they give birth. But *birth is a dynamic process*, which is a way of saying that, for all kinds of reasons, the best laid birth plans sometimes have to be abandoned or adapted during labour – this in itself can be disappointing and even traumatic to any new mum.

Even when birth goes well and as planned, it is a huge physical and emotional event that can take time for mother and baby, and your partner, to process. What is most important is that mother and baby both emerge from the birth safely.

Even if the birth has been traumatic, so long as people around you recognise that fact, you and your baby can recover. People naturally express their concern for the mum after a traumatic birth, which is right. We tend to hope and assume that the baby didn't 'know' because it is too young to be aware. But birth can be a shock and a trauma for the baby too, especially if interventions took place during birth that stopped, or stopped short, some of the natural stages of delivery. There may well be two traumatised people, mother and baby – it is helpful to recognise this.

So what can we do? Let's consider several different groups of births: those born by planned C-section, emergency C-section, difficult but mother and baby are still together, difficult and baby in SCBU.

Birth by planned C-section babies

Planned C-section babies are at less risk than the other groups as mum is prepared and has a good idea about what's coming. Mothers now have the option of having 'a natural caesarean' which allows you more say in the delivery, in terms of the atmosphere in the delivery room, and also aims for minimal physical contact between doctor and baby during delivery. If all goes according to plan, this may make the birth very satisfying for the mother. However, we do know that many, though not all, C-section babies are restless and irritable. If we think of the trauma of coming fast from a warm safe place inside the womb, to the stark cold reality of the delivery room, we can empathise. Everyone is happy about the safe arrival and it may be hard to think about what the experience may have been like for the baby. It is helpful if you can maintain the *symbiotic relationship* for as long as possible, in as relaxed an environment as is possible, with mum and baby allowed to maintain that closeness that they had, until the baby is relaxed and at ease. This is why midwives often encourage 'skin-to-skin' contact between mother and baby, and father and baby, at birth. This helps your family feel close, and will actually provide physiological help to the baby, as they recover from birth.

> *'Skin-to-skin contact helps the baby to adjust to life outside the womb and is highly important for supporting mothers to initiate breastfeeding and to develop a close, loving relationship with their baby through restful sleep and easy feeding plus the establishment of a routine of eat and sleep.'*
> Unicef

If, for whatever reason, mum cannot have this contact immediately after birth, or needs support to have it, it is important that the relationship between mum and baby is 'held' by someone else, rather than the baby being taken over by another. It is tempting for others to say they will help by taking care of the baby. It is understandable that mum will be grateful for this offer, but it is best for baby if the close relationship with mum is maintained. So mum holds the baby and partner holds mum, rather than passing the baby to the partner.

Birth by emergency C-section

Emergency C-sections can be very traumatic for mother and child. They only happen when the baby is distressed, or the physical health of the mother is in danger. This means that the potential of death has been brought into the experience of both mother and baby. This is a huge fear for the parents and, of course, the newborn has no way of processing that fear. The same response is needed, in keeping mother and child in the symbiotic relationship until a routine is established, but it can be harder to do. The mother will inevitably have to process strong feelings of fear of losing her child and her own life, as well as, potentially, anger at the child for putting her through such fear. It is impossible for the mother to express these thoughts and feelings without fear of judgement from her partner, grandparents and others, so mothers may keep these feelings hidden. These hidden feelings can turn to guilt and depression and a sense of not being good enough. This, in turn, can have a serious impact on your relationship with your baby.

It is very important to acknowledge and 'allow' the feelings when this happens. You can recover from these feelings if you and others face them. In this way your relationship with your baby can grow in a healthy way, which will be vital for your baby's sense of self.

Difficult births – mother and baby still together

A prolonged and painful delivery though the vagina can have other effects. There may be physical damage to the mum which will have an impact on the relationship with their partner; this can

> **These days, mothers and babies are often expected to be up and about instantly after the birth, and to post positive pictures of themselves on social media and to family. There is often not enough consideration of the impact that the birth has had, and that it takes time to settle and process the experience afterwards. Supporting mum to support baby is what is needed, allowing her to say 'I need time before I rejoin the world'**

lead to resentment which, again, can be very difficult to admit or talk about. The effort of the delivery can leave mother and child exhausted, making it hard for them to come together in a positive way.

These days, mothers and babies are often expected to be up and about instantly after the birth, and to post positive pictures of themselves on social media and to family. There is often not enough consideration of the impact that the birth has had, and that it takes time to settle and process the experience afterwards. Again, acknowledging your feelings will help. Hiding them is usually destructive. But they need to be processed away from the baby if possible so that it is not carrying the mother's anguish from the beginning. Supporting mum to support baby is what is needed, allowing her to say 'I need time before I rejoin the world'. Unhelpfully, mums can be competitive about who had the 'worst' or 'best' delivery; avoid getting involved in this – it can build up pressure and resentment which is harmful to your relationship with your baby.

Difficult births – mother and baby separated (Special Care Baby Unit)

Sometimes, things go wrong during birth and a baby has to go to the special care baby unit (SCBU) for lifesaving care. Their stay in SCBU may be brief or prolonged. If brief, the impact is likely to be similar to the emergency C-section. However, prolonged stays bring a whole range of other issues.

Babies in SCBU may be there because they are premature, they have a recognised disabling condition, the birth was so strenuous that they need help to breathe and eat, or they were injured in the process through lack of oxygen or something else. All the reasons they are there are likely to be alarming. Seeing needles and tubes being put into your tiny baby is likely to be shocking, and can even seem barbaric. You will likely feel helpless and extremely anxious, apart from which you yourself will be struggling to process your own birth experience – you will yourself be in shock at all that has happened and is happening. Medical and nursing staff can be emotionally challenged as well as parents and wider family. There will usually be a delay before parents and child can be reunited and then only through the sides of a special cot.

> " A mother's feelings can be very extreme and unexpected in these circumstances …I have heard a mother say that she sat and prayed for her child to live and then, when it did, wished that it hadn't when she knew how disabled it was. But she couldn't say that and carried those feelings alone for many years.

The trauma is obvious but the healing for a parent may not come purely as a result of their child's life being saved. It is more complicated than this. A mother's feelings can be very extreme and unexpected in these circumstances, and may be contradictory and confusing. Many mothers feel shame about their feelings and instinctively try to hide them, which makes them feel more isolated, and means their feelings have 'nowhere to go'. I have heard a mother say that she sat and prayed for her child to live and then, when it did, wished that it hadn't when she knew how disabled it was. But she couldn't say that and carried those feelings alone for many years.

To give mother and child the best chance in life we have to face the trauma for both of them. We must ensure that they have an opportunity to grow together and that comes from first establishing and/or preserving the symbiotic relationship.

The effect of birth on the symbiotic relationship

As we saw in Chapter 1, Mahler and her colleagues describe the symbiotic relationship as a sense of mother and child still being one or joined. Winnicott (1964; 1992), another recognized pioneer in infant mental health, refers to this closeness as an essential part of the child's start in life. The word *symbiosis* means 'joined for mutual benefit' and that is the best way to think of it. Both parent and child benefit from that closeness being established.

The benefits of skin-to-skin contact

When symbiosis is proving difficult the baby will be fractious and the mother anxious, and it becomes increasingly difficult to work out which came first. We do know that if this is not addressed it gets worse. Probably the most effective approach is for mum to lie down with the baby on her chest in close contact with her heartbeat.

The benefits of skin-to-skin contact after birth

There is a growing body of evidence that skin-to-skin contact after the birth helps babies and their mothers in many ways.
- Calms and relaxes both mother and baby.
- Regulates the baby's heart rate and breathing, helping them to better adapt to life outside the womb.
- Stimulates digestion and an interest in feeding.
- Regulates temperature.
- Enables colonisation of the baby's skin with the mother's friendly bacteria, thus providing protection against infection.
- Stimulates the release of hormones to support breastfeeding and mothering.
- Improves oxygen saturation.

- Reduces cortisol (stress) levels particularly following painful procedures.
- Encourages pre-feeding behaviour.
- Assists with growth.
- May reduce hospital stay.
- If the mother expresses following a period of skin-to-skin contact, her milk volume will improve and the milk expressed will contain the most up-to-date antibodies.

Unicef (2019): www.unicef.org.uk/babyfriendly/baby-friendly-resources/implementing-standards-resources/skin-to-skin-contact/

Having this contact with your baby should have benefits for you, too, but it is important that you are as calm as you can be – you will have a more relaxed heartbeat if you are not hungry or worried about practicalities or visitors, need the toilet and so on. It is up to everyone around you to make sure you are feeling supported and looked after.

Winnicott refers to the need for the father's initial task being to support the mother so she can look after the child. In modern times it may not be the father but another trusted adult. What matters is that someone does it. It may take some time but if the mother and child can stay peacefully like that until the baby is completely relaxed there will be lots of benefits. This is just as true for the mother and child where all went smoothly during birth. Establishing the symbiotic relationship

The symbiotic stage lasts only a few weeks but is the foundation of everything that follows. The baby that struggles to feed, that remains fractious, that cannot have physical contact with mum will be changed by those experiences. If we consider that the baby has no resources for processing what is happening we can envisage the extreme fear that it may experience and, when we hear distressed crying, the rage that follows. Fear and anger are closely linked. Melanie Klein (1975) referred to the murderous rage of the newborn baby who is powerless to make things right. Sadly, we can find adults with a similar frame of mind. This suggests a failure in their lives to establish a joining-together with another human being.

Happily, most babies get through this stage with no serious mishaps. It will be different for every one, including identical twins – the beginnings of the future formed personality are already set. The failure to make meaningful contact will almost certainly lead to relationship issues. The establishment of a happy healthy contact will enable your child to get to the next stage. If all has gone well with the delivery it should be fairly easy to establish the symbiotic relationship. However, establishing a good feeding routine can take a little while. The core issue will always be trust. So long as the baby can trust that food will be there when needed and is provided with emotional warmth then the relationship will develop.

'A baby is born with a need to be loved – and never outgrows it.'
Frank

Chapter 3: Feeling Their Way – Differentiation

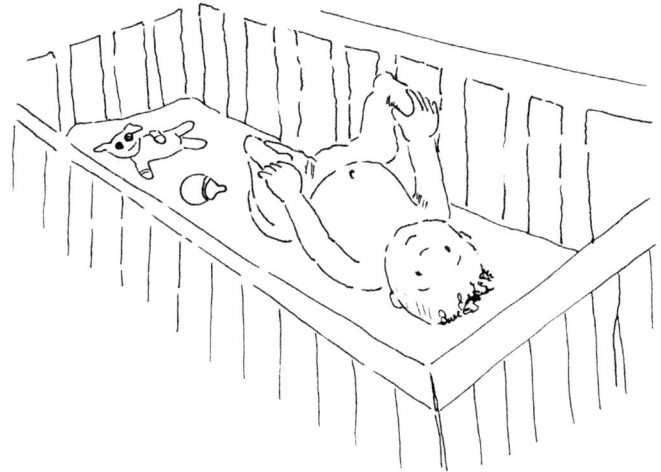

'This little piggy went to market, this little piggy stayed at home…'

What does differentiation 'look like'?

Mahler referred to the next stage of emotional development as *differentiation*. This stage typically lasts from a few weeks to about nine or ten months. It is possible that this stage is when you might notice the first signs of behaviour that is not typical or 'ordinary'. But equally it may also be that at this stage a parent/carer might look at behaviour that is actually quite 'normal' and think that something is wrong – this may lead to a change in the way the parent or carer behaves around the baby.

This is the stage when the baby starts to explore its own body and the world around it. The baby is very egocentric and has no interest in anything much other than getting its own needs met. It follows that, even though they may spend quite long periods happily gurgling in their cot, they will soon protest if they need food or a clean nappy. All their behaviours are what is called *self-referenced* – all about them – things like looking at their feet and hands, exploring the sides of the cot or pram, chewing on a teat instead of sucking, presumably testing the limits of their abilities.

To help your baby move through this stage, you and your baby's other primary carers need to be available and responsive. Feeling secure with his/her primary carers, your baby will continue to develop and explore their physical environment. They will respond with a smile but only look for attention, usually through crying, to get a physical need met. When your baby is with someone they feel secure around, they will be relaxed and develop. If they don't feel secure, they may start engaging in what are called *compensation behaviours* – if a baby realizes that their needs are met, they may stop asking. This actually slows down the development of their personality. This is sometimes described as *blunting*, where the joy of being alive becomes tempered with the uncertainty of what will happen next. If this happens, some babies will become more demanding as they cannot recognise and trust that their needs will be met.

If you give a baby positive feedback on feeding, pooing, smiling and so on they will know that they are valued and acceptable. If a parent or carer responds in a negative way to these things, the baby may start to be wary and respond differently. Children who experience other more obvious trauma at this age will also be affected, and later behaviours are likely to reflect that trauma.

Problems with the symbiotic relationship that show at the differentiation stage

Babies' brains are growing very quickly during this period – so, even babies who have struggled to establish a symbiotic relationship with a parent/primary carer will still move to some extent into the differentiation stage, because of that neurological development. But those babies may show less interest in themselves or their surroundings. If you notice this, it may be an early warning sign to a parent or those people supporting them to take action to help establish better bonds and closeness. It can be easier to think that it's 'a good baby' that is quite happy to be alone, but in fact that *isn't* a good sign. *A baby who seems to have given up on adults in the first few months of life needs help.*

Babies who were always likely to find it hard because of difficult birth circumstances will need help too, but if they have managed to reach a good symbiotic relationship they should do well. Babies with serious mental impairment through brain damage or other conditions will also need help. They can be guided to explore their hands and feet and surroundings. They may be more sleepy, and there is a risk that they will be left to sleep, but they need stimulation to wake them up emotionally as well as physically.

'Every day, in a 100 small ways, our children ask, 'Do you hear me? Do

you see me? Do I matter?' Their behavior often reflects our response.'
L.R. Knost

It may be that a poorly baby who cries a lot is trying to make contact and needs to be held. Equally, it may be that the poorly child who doesn't cry is so traumatised by their injury that they are in shock and can't cry.

The differentiation stage can be enjoyable, with lots of cuddles, a pattern of food and sleep, joy in being alive. Children who get stuck at this stage and don't go on to develop relationship skills may go on to grow up emotionally flat and wary of people.

Gazing at your baby

A key aspect of this stage is referred to by Winnicott as *reverie*, where the baby sees itself reflected in its mother's eyes. A baby at this age will gaze at its mother's/carer's face with apparent concentration. It is important that the mother has the time to gaze back at them. Winnicott described the process of a baby seeing itself reflected and so 'confirmed':

- The baby who sees love and positive feelings will grow emotionally.
- The baby who sees hostility will withdraw.
- The baby whose mother can't look at him/her will stop developing as there is no feedback.

> **'Feeling connected to other people is probably the deepest satisfaction we will ever know. How terrible for children who are being brought up without that capacity'**
> **Sue Gerhardt**

Sadly, sometimes when a mother suffers from post-natal depression, she may find she cannot bear to look at her child. In this situation it is really important that the baby's other care givers and the people who support them step in to make sure the baby is getting the connection that it is looking for.

'The false self'

Winnicott had a theory about the development of a 'false self' – this is how he described what happens when a baby/small child feels unacceptable to their mother/primary carer. Winnicott observed that the child would then develop patterns of behaviour that are more acceptable to their carer, and – even at this age – suppress its true nature. We meet many adults who have done this, unconsciously, and who only get in touch with their true nature during therapy.

Chapter 4:
Learning Fast – Practising

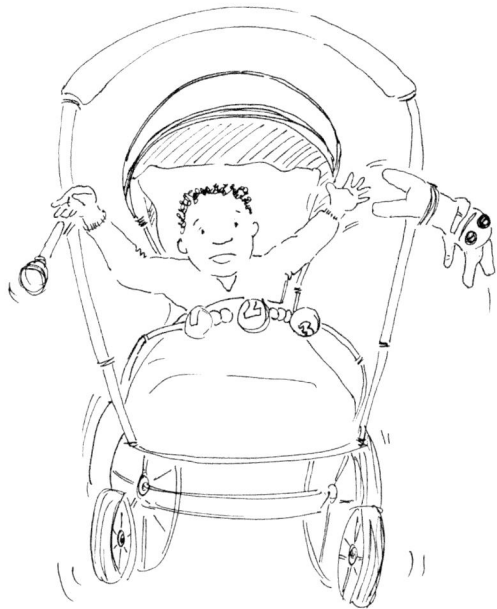

'Children learn as they play. Most importantly, in play children learn how to learn.'
O Fred Donaldson

As the brain grows so quickly, a baby becomes able to do more and more things and learn new skills. When they find they can do something new, they will do it again and again until they realise they can do more and more, and move on to the next thing. Mahler called this *practising*, to describe the way it looks as though the child is practising a new skill until it is good at it, and then just adds it to a list of skills that it already has. The first 'skill' is usually rolling over and most of us have seen babies rolling over and over, but then losing interest as they become able to shuffle or crawl.

The practising stage can be fun as there is a lot of development happening. Rolling over, sitting up, throwing things, grasping things, then shuffling and crawling are all the milestones that need to be reached. These are physical skills that come naturally. Sounds become available too, and gurgling then babbling follow. Parents and carers should notice and respond to all of these things to make sure they are maintained and progressed through. Children do not develop in a vacuum; they need feedback and encouragement so the skills develop in the context of a warm and loving relationship. It is important that children feel they have your full attention. It is sad to see so many children ignored as their parent is glued to a screen, or given a screen instead of attention.

> **Children do not develop in a vacuum; they need feedback and encouragement so the skills develop in the context of a warm and loving relationship.**

Repetitive behaviours – getting stuck

Some children may become 'stuck' on these *repetitive behaviours*; this might be because they are on the autistic spectrum, or have another obsessive or ritualistic condition. Research suggests that people with these conditions are emotionally stuck at the practising stage. We cannot prove this, but clinically I have many examples of older children and adults with these conditions who have early trauma in their history. We also see clinical examples of people who make progress in their tolerance of disorder when treated at this emotional level.

Sue Gerhardt's book *Why Love Matters* (2004) explains the brain's – or 'cognitive' – changes that can be shown by neuroscience when children don't get the emotional nurture they need when they are very young. Put simply, without attention, engagement, love and affection, a child's brain doesn't develop as quickly or in the same way as it does with them. This suggests that helping a child to get through the practising stage to the next one is vitally important, and may reduce the incidence and extent of autism and promote healthy emotional development. Some research indicates better long term outcomes for children who show early signs of autism when parents get better support and guidance.

> **Put simply, without attention, engagement, love and affection, a child's brain doesn't develop as quickly or in the same way as it does with them.**

When things go wrong

There are lots of reasons why this stage can go wrong. A child with a disability or with early trauma will not necessarily progress from differentiation to practising without help. If there seems to be no sign of progress by ten months it is time to look into what is happening and try to help the child progress. Again, the presence of the mother/primary carer (also referred to as the 'key attachment figure' or 'significant other'), is vital. This adult needs to notice what the child can do, which may be as simple as poking its tongue out, then reflect the behaviour back with a smile and encouraging noises; gradually, the response is shaped into something more developed. Similarly with reaching out a hand – this may be an unconscious movement but you are trying to make it conscious by drawing attention to the ability. Once you have established a conscious behaviour, the baby can build on it, and this can happen with profoundly disabled children as well. Children need to be encouraged to practise a behaviour until it morphs into a new one and so on. It is intensive interaction and needs to be part of the whole adult/child relationship, not just some sessions now and then. You are, effectively, waking up the emotional side of the child that has become frozen in response to trauma.

Taking trauma seriously

Children who have experienced something that is personally traumatic for them in the first year of life may enter the practising stage but be unable to get across it without help. The longer it takes for them to get that help, the more stuck the behaviour becomes because brain development slows down because of it. It is very important that early signs are noticed. Most parents will be told to 'wait and see' if they report concerns about repetitive behaviour and detachment in a one-year-old. My wish is that parents are offered guidance on what to do.

The first thing to accept is that these repetitive behaviours are neurotypical for the 10 to 15-month-old child, who will repeat something over and over. They will study intently something that they notice. They will be totally absorbed and take no notice of others. They will self-soothe as if not expecting any help. These behaviours are fine if present some of the time. If present all of the time they are a warning sign that something has happened to cause fear and mistrust, and they are transferring their trust in people to trust in the certainty of objects. The best way to approach this is to take the child back to the previous stage and provide the same eye-gazing closeness of the differentiation stage, the warmth of contact and the certainty of being available. It can be easier to have a child who occupies itself but it is not setting a good developmental path if they do it too soon. It is really hard to hear a mum say what a good baby they have because it is not demanding and occupies itself, when it is clearly too young to be doing that.

> *'Since the earliest period of our life was preverbal, everything depended on emotional interaction. Without someone to reflect our emotions, we had no way of knowing who we were'*
> (John Bradshaw, 2006)

Older children and adults

Older children and adults who are emotionally stuck at this stage will often have been given diagnoses of autism, ADHD, severe challenging behaviour, OCD, and some of the personality disorders. Often the cognitive development has continued, but it may be impaired by emotional issues. When there is a mismatch between the emotional and cognitive stage it is clear that the parent/carer and child may need more support. The plan is to enable the emotional development to progress and so allow the cognitive self to become more effective. Once the cognitive self, the reasoning self, is working properly, life gets better. The next stage will look at the move towards reasoning.

Chapter 5: Give and Take – Early Rapprochement

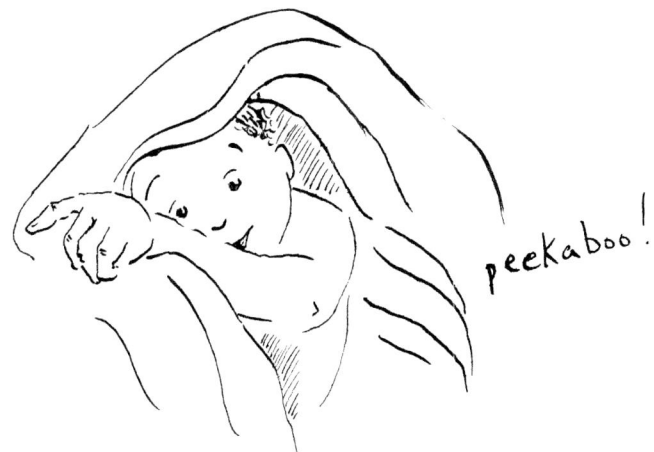

'Round and round the garden / Like a teddy bear / One step, two step / Tickle you under there!'

As the practising stage progresses, a child becomes able to speak and walk. Once they can do that, they can say 'no' and they can run away. So begins the stage of two-way interaction – talking to each other. The relationship between carer and child changes – it isn't just a case of the adult meeting the child's needs, but one where both of your needs become important. Mother/carer and child are involved in an emotional dance, both wanting their decisions to be the ones that hold sway, and both motivated to make it happen – in other words, you want what you want, and the child wants what they want!

This is the stage when we often start confronting or arguing with the child; it can be hard not to do this, but it is usually not helpful. If, as the adult, you are trying to 'win' and shut down argument, your child isn't learning to negotiate or compromise. This should be the beginning of the well-known 'win-win' negotiating that we hear about in management skills. But the adult needs to take the lead. It's an exciting developmental period, with rapid development of physical as well as emotional skills. The stage lasts from approximately 15 months to 24 months, with individual variations. It is easy to see when the child moves on to the next stage, if their relationship with their main carer continues throughout.

No you can't, yes I can

In this stage the child believes it can do more than it can, so needs protecting from over stretching, but encouraging to try new things – this is a delicate balance and we can't expect to get it right all the time. There will be tantrums and embarrassing moments when the child throws themselves on the supermarket floor, especially if a new baby has arrived by now. The arrival of a sibling is often traumatising for the older child. They have been the centre of attention for two years and suddenly they are not. As the new baby will actually need less attention at first (although, see Chapter 2 on symbiosis), it is worth investing in the two-year-old and helping them to progress through the *rapprochement* stage. A crucial part of this is to enhance awareness of the world, so always saying what is happening and what will happen next helps with this.

> **In this stage the child believes it can do more than it can, so needs protecting from over stretching, but encouraging to try new things – this is a delicate balance and we can't expect to get it right all the time.**

For example, in the morning, going to the cot saying 'we're going to get up, have a wash and dress, then make breakfast'. Then, during breakfast, say, 'We're nearly finished so time to clean teeth and then we can play' or whatever fits with the day's activities. This keeps the child engaged and interested, as well as both parties staying fully committed to each other. It is generally not helpful to get into disputes with children at this stage as they revert quickly to a more primitive omnipotence and demand whatever it is they take a fancy to. They have been used to their significant other knowing what they need without asking, so they cannot tolerate, initially, that things have changed, or be aware that it is they who has changed. It can be very confusing for parents and caregivers too as this very agreeable baby changes into a tyrant almost overnight. In addition to this, there is teething to contend with as well, pain that cannot be explained nor understood. Add the first cold or sore throat and the world begins to look and feel like a very scary place.

Needless to say, this is a very critical stage of development and the majority of very complex adults that I have worked with have been stuck at this stage. Often the trauma is a new sibling, associated with mum leaving to go to hospital, so there is a separation to manage as well. Sometimes it is more serious, with permanent loss of the significant other for all sorts of reasons. Adoption at this stage needs very careful handling. Children are likely to shut down emotionally as a defence against their fear and appear to be accepting the new order of things, whereas they can go into a 'waiting state' that lasts for a very long time, and sometimes forever if it is not noticed. Children will respond differently to trauma depending on how stable their lives were before. If everything had been going smoothly before, then the reaction is likely to be noticed and, hopefully, the child can be helped to process the event. If things were already a bit rocky then the event will be processed as proof that the world is not safe and the psychological consequences will be more severe, leading to a different life trajectory than was expected.

Potty training

Potty training becomes a part of this stage and can highlight and intensify a lot of the behaviours you are already seeing – potty training is an opportunity for your child to do as you say i.e. to be compliant, or try to take control, or get comfort. If parents don't listen to the signs from their child or manage the process consistently and well, or if there have been issues earlier, there can be a range of problems including children refusing to poo in the potty, or getting constipated, or deliberately pooing in the wrong place at the wrong time.

Moving to the next stage

If all is well and there is little or no trauma then there will be relatively smooth transition to late rapprochement. If there is some trauma but it is processed well, a child might actually gain some resilience at this stage. Older children and adults who have continued to progress cognitively but got stuck emotionally at the stage of early rapprochement are likely to be diagnosed as emotionally unstable or be troubled by addictive behaviour, including eating disorders. These conditions may often be a response to the recognition that the world is grey, and not black and white. The seeking of certainty for these individuals becomes crucial, and maladaptive behaviour develops in an unconscious attempt to find the line that is certain. Sadly, the emotional pain is so big that most offers to help are pushed away. It takes determination and consistency to make a difference and build trust. It can be done so long as the size of the task is recognised and the parameters can be put in place.

Most children progress gradually from this stage to late rapprochement. This is where the see-saw tips from the adult taking the lead to a more equal state of affairs, with the child initiating things and becoming able to negotiate, using developing cognitive skills and showing what they can do. The first signs of this next stage of development are likely to be them hesitating, or thinking in a situation where before they have reacted with frustration.

Chapter 6: Moving Away – Late Rapprochement

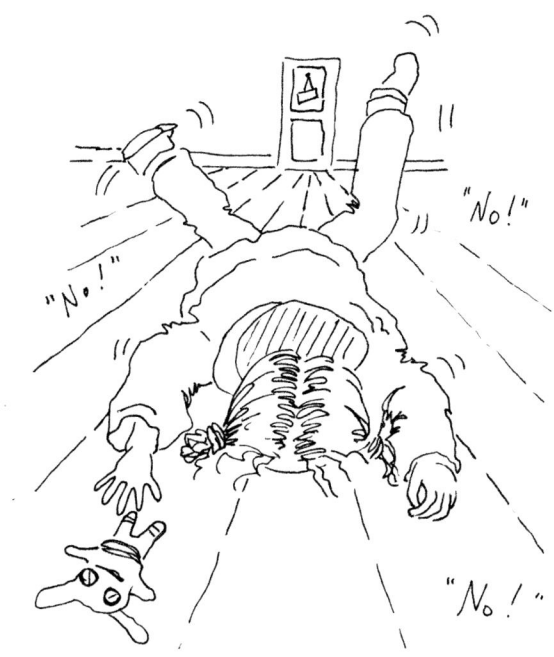

'Your child will eventually be able to leave you, knowing they can always return and will be loved, and cared for.'
John Bowlby

It ain't what you do, it's the way that you do it

As a child progresses through their second year and approaches the age of three, they grow – physically, and in terms of their identity. They become more confident in two-way activities, show signs of being able to respond to reason, and can understand 'if-then' situations.

Example
'If we put the toys away, then we can have ice cream' – this suggests that cooperation can have a positive outcome, as opposed to: 'You had better put the toys away or there will be no ice-cream' – this reinforces that the adult has all the power and control, to take something away before it has even been given.

The positive 'if-then' approach is still about working together and means that your child experiences support rather than criticism. It's also important that the child is not expected to do more than it can. If a false self (see Chapter 3) has started to develop at an earlier stage, it will become strengthened and set in this stage as more thinking becomes available. The child will start to work out how to be acceptable to the parent and patterns of behaviour will become set. Sometimes this will mean that the child is trying to do things in a way that meets their parents' own psychological needs, rather than their own. So, for example, the parent who feels unloved by other adults may expect more love from their child. The child will be unable to meet this need but may find a way to look as though they can in order to protect themselves, and then end up denying their own needs. Children who become prematurely independent at this stage may do quite well for some time but are likely to carry with them some emotional pain.

It is vital that parents are able to give the child room to develop independence, and encouragement, without forcing it. Find times when you can share decision making with your child – even about simple things, such as how to fix a toy – this will help them to start thinking about how to solve problems. It is best to find a balance between too much and too little help. Being able to guide the child through the stage is a privilege, and fun, too, when all is going well.

Making transitions

Children are often starting nursery or are with a childminder at this stage, and may be having care from different adults. They can usually manage this alright so long as they can be aware of the limits and are clear about when they will see you again. Winnicott advised that children often need a transitional object. This is an item that provides security in the absence of their significant care giver. It is often referred to as a 'security blanket' and can be anything from an actual blanket to a toy or a teddy. It is whatever the child loves and feels it needs.

Most 'neurotypical' children will pass through this stage before their fourth birthday. It is usually easy to see whether or not a child is doing well at this stage. Signs that they are having difficulties include little or no initiation of games or conversations, difficulty with making decisions (within their expected level), lack of interaction, lack of independent functioning, again 'within reasonable levels'.

A child may seem to be 'too independent' if the independence comes from a sense of fear or a false self. But every child is different and many of the traits are positive, and simply signs of their developing character.

Trauma and recovery can be character building and provide a whole range of skills that lead to a productive and fulfilling life. It makes for the richness of the human experience. And most of the time all will be well.

At this stage it begins to be possible and useful to start using rewards to shape children's behaviour or make it more likely that they will behave positively.

If you try to use a reward system too soon it can be counter-productive, and actually cause the child to behave worse. So, for example, if you give sweets as a reward for children to do as they are asked, you may quickly find yourself in a situation where the child behaves badly *until* they get sweets, rather than to behave well to get them. When parents/carers and child are close and know each other well, this process is easier.

Chapter 7: Knowing Me, Knowing You – Making it to Individuation

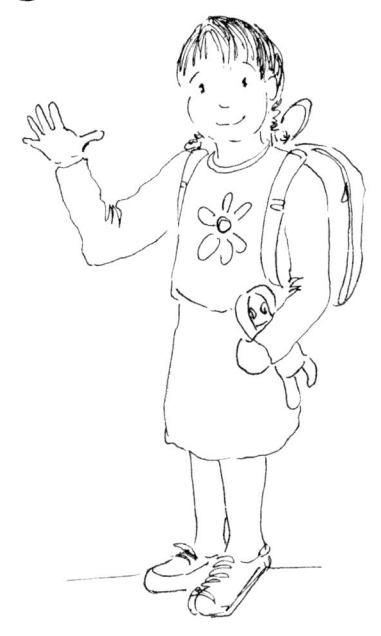

'If children feel safe, they can take risks, ask questions, make mistakes, learn to trust, share their feelings, and grow.'
Alfie Kohn

Finding the right balance

If all goes well and the a child has progressed through the stages well enough, then they will reach a stage of being able to be separate from the primary carer with what is called 'manageable anxiety'. This is known as *individuation*. This is not a stage in which the child has *no* anxiety – a certain amount of anxiety helps children to be wary and cautious, which is important to keep them safe. A child with no anxiety is at risk of being reckless and may be vulnerable. At the same time, a child who expects someone else to solve any problems they have will also have problems. Autistic children are often observed to expect an external source to solve their problems. They may lack that internal model of the world that would allow them to make judgements about what is safe or what to do next. This is also noticeable in other children who, on one hand, have needed to be too independent too soon and, on the other hand, who have been overprotected and not allowed to experiment with growing independence.

It is not a 'given' that all children will reach the individuation stage; there are many adults who are functioning well enough who have not fully individuated. They are cognitively able enough to manage their world with what we call *intellectual defences* – they rationalise anything that causes them anxiety and label it in a way that is acceptable to them. So, for example, someone with a phobia which links to an early trauma, of which they have no memory, will say to themselves, and to others 'I've always been the same so I've got used to it'. Others will only be able to function well if they are in a close reliable relationship, so will always look to have one, and so may have relationships that aren't good for them just so they can feel connected.

> *'We don't have to get it right all the time, we just need to be good enough.'*
> DW Winnicott (1971)

Winnicott talks about *'good enough parenting'* and this term emphasises that meeting every need a child expresses can be as harmful as not meeting any, or very few – dealing with frustration is part of growing up. Coping with what you don't like, accepting 'no' and learning to share are all part of these early stages.

We look for synchronicity between physical, cognitive and emotional development. If they are all in tune with each other all will be well enough. When they are not, the signs of distress become observable. The worst-case scenario is the psychopath who has a well-developed cognitive self, but is emotionally an omnipotent egocentric baby. The cognitive self will use all its power to satisfy the primitive needs. The child with an intellectual disability will have delayed cognitive development but may not have delayed emotional development. If there is delayed or arrested emotional development they will lack the cognitive skills to hide it and distressed behaviour will be evident. This group comprises the majority of the detained ID group, detained in full-time education or specialist secure facilities.

In his book *'The Child, the Family and the Outside World'* (1964; 1992) Winnicott describes the processes of progressing from being in the very close relationship with one person, to relating to the wider family group, and then progressing on to relating to the wider world of school and friendships. This book was written many years ago and still carries real words of wisdom. Mahler *et al*'s work gives us a description of behaviours to look for at the different stages, and hence provides us with an early warning system. It is hoped that the above will help to make some of these ideas more accessible to more people.

Chapter 8: Finding Support – What Happens When Things Go Wrong?

Sadly, very few infant support staff will be familiar with the development of the emotional self. Traditional services concentrate on physical milestones and then social skills. These are linked, but the underlying emotional development is more subtle and therefore not as obvious. It is also not easy to think of little babies being traumatised. There are some positive developments: it is now fully recognised and accepted that tiny babies in incubators need physical contact and that they can experience pain, so hopefully some of those traumas will be reduced. However, the level of midwife and health visitor support is much reduced nowadays and they are unlikely to receive specialist training in this area. We need always to remember that parenthood is a job for life for which we receive little or no training and there are no qualifications to secure in advance. We know more than we used to and it is hoped that, in time, all staff training will include this extra information and all prospective parents will have access to it too.

It has become usual practice for mothers to identify a birth partner; a positive development might be if we were to look for a support partner for the first few years. It can be lonely raising a child and many mums feel inadequate and challenged. They can also feel rejected by professionals who don't give a useful response to concerns. This will usually be because the concerns are outside of the expertise of the person rather than a lack of interest, but it doesn't help.

Adults who are raising children who are not their own have additional problems. Often these will be grandchildren or other family members and, sometimes, non-familial adoptions. Children removed from their mothers at birth are usually fostered first, leading to them having to bond with one person and then another. They don't always do this very well and it would be worth exploring if this would work better if the new mother were to try to start again with establishing the symbiotic relationship first.

What happens when things go wrong?

Throughout this booklet I have used examples of *indicators* when things are not quite as we would like, and there is the potential for trauma to have an impact on the developing child. There is a whole wealth of information about childhood mental health issues and usually these are addressed medically or within models that have evolved over many years. The model described in this book has not been widely accepted but is gathering more credence over time. It may be that birth and early trauma has been too painful to recognise. It may be the resistance to psychodynamic ideas that are hard to test. However, the ability to observe behaviour associated with emotional developmental stages helps to make the progression testable. This approach has been used with children and adults with intellectual disabilities for some years now and is proving to be useful.

Studies of adults with seriously complex behaviour has led to some tentative conclusions about the consequences of being stuck emotionally at the different stages. Some of these have been described here.

When people get 'stuck'

It is rare to find an adult stuck at the *symbiotic stage* but it is possible to find adults who have no attachments at all, who put no value on human interaction. The implication is that they never had a primary attachment and have grown up in emotional isolation. They are unable to form relationships and are emotionally flat. There is some evidence of this in the orphans that are found around the world, as well as individuals we see in mental health facilities, prisons and homeless hostels. They can seek and accept practical physical help but have no ability to show gratitude or other emotions. This makes them difficult to help sometimes and it is rarely recognised that they have been traumatised from a very early age.

It is more common to find people stuck at the *differentiation stage*. They will have complex unstable relationships with people, may have diagnoses of severe mental ill-health such as schizophrenia or psychotic depression, or sociopathic personality disorder. These are the individuals who had the beginnings of an attachment and secure relationship that then went wrong, and became complicated. It is very often missed at the time. It is the one-person level of emotional development that has not progressed beyond that and the person cannot, therefore, function in relationships.

Individuals stuck at the *practising stage* have been described to some extent. There are many conditions where the behaviour is help-seeking, or certainty-seeking, repetitive and focused on achieving the unachievable. So many of the addictions, to food, gambling, sex and such like, fall into this category, as well as autism, obsessive compulsive disorder, bipolar disorder and others. The conditions all require external input to help, as the individual lacks the internal resources to resolve their problems themselves. It may be that the brain changes from early childhood cannot be recovered from; however, clinical evidence suggests that establishing meaningful attachments can enable some progress to be made towards trust and internal locus of control, with a realistic appraisal of what is achievable. This then leads to a level of acceptance and contentment with life as it is, and the driven, obsessive behaviour diminishes.

The *early rapprochement stage* is a time of rapid change. It is the time when trust and two-way interaction comes into play. The 'dance' of this stage is played out clearly in emotionally unstable personality disorder (formerly known as borderline personality disorder). A small child who demands something and then rejects it can be seen as amusing. The adult who does the same is seen as problematic. The constant testing and inability to manage frustration is characteristic of this condition and no amount of appealing to reason helps until a close trusting relationship can be established. A core issue is to help support staff not to take rejection personally and to be prepared for the rejection that follows something positive. It seems as though a positive few hours activates the fear of loss and leads to the loss being precipitated before it comes. These individuals suffer serious distress and often end up in care settings where less is expected of them and they can attach to the place instead of the people. The old long-stay hospitals were safe places for this group in terms of maintaining an existence. If a therapeutic intervention is to help people to progress to a better way of life, it needs careful individual provision with safe and reliable people present at all times. Increasing the tolerance of separation then leads to progress to a more mature state.

Depression and anxiety are linked to *late rapprochement*. The child who graduates to this stage is beginning to trust in the world and to make some decisions, based on understanding. If those decisions go wrong then the seeds are sown for later difficulties. And, of course, the decisions may have been unrealistic. The two-year-old who says to themselves they are pleased a new baby is here, then finds themselves overwhelmed with anger and hatred, will become confused and doubt their ability to get it right, and so with the conflict that may arise with potty training. Feeling unacceptable and rejected for getting it wrong can have lasting consequences. Most depressed and anxious people have clear ideas about what upsets them. Tracing this back can usually arrive at the events that underpin it. Sadly, it has usually been going on for years before it is explored in therapy, and has become reinforced by other events, making it slow work sometimes to make it better. Symptom control with medication is often useful.

Adults wanting to explore this themselves can try a technique described by Karen Horney (1994). You start with something that has caused distress recently, then ask yourself when was the last time you felt like this, then the time before and so on until you get as far back as you can. It may take a few sessions and may be worth writing out a timeline of your life with key events on it to start with, adding others as they are recalled. Not everyone can get to the actual events that took place before the age of three, but getting close can usually help to clarify what the initial fear was, and then work out how it has been compounded since.

Epilogue: Some Words of Reassurance

The purpose of this book is to be helpful and reassuring. Most children do well enough most of the time. Most people benefit from negative experiences by becoming more resilient. Most parents do their best. But some babies are hard to 'get going' – they may be fractious from the beginning and consequently cause their parents a great deal of anxiety and distress. The optimistic message here is that there are things that help and make a difference.

Identifying the process of your child's emotional development must be helpful. Many parents will do it intuitively. Others will find one child responds and another doesn't, which is confusing. We are all different and, although the birth experience may have felt the same for the mother, each child will respond to it in its own way.

> *'If there is one thing developmental psychologists have learned over the years, it is that parents don't have to be brilliant psychologists to succeed. They don't have to be supremely gifted teachers… parents just have to be good enough. They have to provide their kids with stable and predictable rhythms. They need to establish the secure emotional bonds that kids can fall back upon in the face of stress.'*
> David Brooks

The most exciting part for me is that we know we can help at whatever stage intervention is offered. Once the issue has been identified it is possible to recreate the emotional nurture that is needed to encourage or promote further development. My early experience was of people with disabilities whose behaviour didn't change for years. I know now that similar people can change if their emotional needs are met. Then their quality of life improves.

People without disabilities can usually use their cognitive skills to help them to understand what has happened to them, and can then work through their distress in the context of a therapeutic relationship. Sadly, they are often offered only a prescription for medication. This can help in the short term but it doesn't offer the warmth and emotional support that is also needed. Holistic approaches are gaining in acceptance so this should help.

The main message is, *'Let's try and reduce the need for later intervention by putting in place preventative measures through learning how to provide the necessary nurturing environment'*. By providing support to new parents so this reduction can happen, we can identify early if there is a drift from optimal development.

References

Gerhardt S (2004) *Why Love Matters: How affection shapes a baby's brain*. London: Routledge.

Horney, K (1994) *Self-analysis*. London: WW Norton and Co.

Klein M (1975) *Envy and Gratitude*. London: Virago.

Mahler M, Pine F and Bergman A (1975) *The Psychological Birth of the Human Infant: Symbiosis and Individuation*. New York: Basic Books. (Reprinted in 1985, 1992, 2008.)

Winnicott D W (1964) The Child, the Family and the Outside World. London: Pelican.

Quotes

Bradshaw J (2006) *Healing the Shame that Binds You*. Health Communications.

Brooks D (2011) *The Social Animal: The hidden sources of love, character, and achievement.* London: Random House.

Donaldson OF Dr (1993) *Playing By Heart: The vision and practice of belonging*. Health Communications Inc

Montessori M (1998) *Creative Development in the Child: The Montessori Approach, Volume One.*